Copyright 2023

Table of Contents

Acne is a chronic, inflammatory skin condition that causes spots and pimples, especially on the face, shoulders, back, neck, chest, and upper arms.

Acne vulgaris is the medical name for common acne -- the presence of blackheads, whiteheads,and other types of pimples on the skin. The most common spots for breakouts are the face, chest, shoulders, and back. Although mild acne may improve with over-the-counter treatments, more severe forms should be treated by a dermatologist.

1. Pumpkin Bread

Prep Time: 5 Minutes

Cook Time: 1hr 5 Minutes

Serving: 9

Ingredients

- 1 Cup Flour
- 3/4 Teaspoon Baking Soda
- 1/2 Teaspoon Baking Powder
- 1 Teaspoon Cinnamon
- 1/2 Teaspoon Salt
- 1 Teaspoon Pumpkin Pie Spice
- 1/2 Cup Canola Oil
- 1/4 Cup Dark Brown Sugar
- 3/4 Cup Sugar
- 2 Large Eggs
- 1 Teaspoon Vanilla
- 1 Cup Pumpkin Puree not pumpkin pie filling

Instructions

1. Preheat the oven to 350 degrees.
2. In a bowl, whisk together the oil, eggs, pumpkin and vanilla. Stir and then add the sugars.
3. Spray a 9x5" bread pan with nonstick spray.
4. In a large bowl, whisk together the flour, baking soda, spices and salt. Set aside.
5. Dump the dry ingredients on the wet ingredients and switching to a rubber spatula or wooden spoon, gently fold the ingredients together just until a few streaks of flour remain.
6. Pour into a bread pan and bake for 50 minutes or until a toothpick comes out clean. Allow to rest for 5 minutes.
7. At this point, slide a knife around the inside of the pan and carefully turn the bread out into your other hand or onto the cooling rack directly if you are gentle.
8. Place it right side up and allow to cool or be like us and dig in because warm bread is the best!

2. The BEST Pumpkin Chocolate Chip Cookies

Prep Time: 10 Minutes

Cook Time: 12 Minutes

Serving: 3

Ingredients

- 1/2 Cup Butter unsalted and softened
- 1 Cup White Sugar
- 1 Large Egg
- 1 Cup Pumpkin Puree
- 1/2 Teaspoon Vanilla
- 2 Cups Flour
- 2 Teaspoons Baking Powder
- 1/2 Teaspoon Baking Soda
- 1/2 Teaspoon Salt
- 2 Teaspoons Cinnamon
- 1/4 Teaspoon Nutmeg
- 1/4 Teaspoon Ground Ginger
- 1/8 Teaspoon Ground Cloves or up to 1/4 Teaspoon
- 2 Cups Chocolate Chips

Instructions

1. Preheat the oven to 375 degrees.
2. Place a silpat or parchment paper on each cookie sheet.
3. It's very important that you start with softened, not melted butter. Add the butter and sugar to a standing mixer and beat for 2 minutes.
4. Add the egg and beat for 30 seconds.
5. Add the pumpkin and vanilla and mix on low, gradually increasing the speed until smooth.
6. In a separate bowl, whisk together the flour, baking powder, baking soda, salt, cinnamon, nutmeg, ginger and cloves.
7. After thoroughly mixing the dry ingredients, add in the chocolate chips and stir.
8. The flour will help the chocolate chips be evenly distributed throughout the cookie.
9. Add the dry ingredients and chocolate chips to the wet ingredients and mix until just combined.
10. Using a cookie or ice cream scoop, scoop the dough on to cookie sheets and bake for 11-12 minutes or until dry looking on top.
11. Remove from the oven and serve.
12. See notes for storage.

3. Pumpkin Crumb Muffins

Prep Time: 5 Minutes

Cook Time: 25 Minutes

Serving: 9

Ingredients

- 2 Cups Flour
- 1 Teaspoon Baking Soda
- 1/2 Teaspoon Salt
- 2 Teaspoons Cinnamon
- 1 1/2 Teaspoons Pumpkin Pie Spice
- 1/4 Cup Sour Cream
- 1/3 Cup Canola Oil
- 1/4 Cup Buttermilk
- 1/4 Cup Dark Brown Sugar
- 3/4 Cup Sugar
- 2 Large Eggs
- 1 1/3 Cups Canned Pumpkin not pumpkin pie filling
- Crumb Topping
- 1/2 Cup Flour
- 1/4 Cup Sugar

- 5 Tablespoons Brown Sugar
- 1 Teaspoon Cinnamon
- 6 Tablespoons Butter melted
- Powdered Sugar for garnish

Instructions

1. Preheat the oven to 350 degrees.
2. Spray a Jumbo Muffin Pan with nonstick spray.
3. In a large bowl, whisk together the flour, baking soda, spices and salt. Set aside.
4. In another bowl, whisk together the oil, sour cream, buttermilk and sugars. Add in the eggs and whisk again, but be sure to not over mix.
5. Dump the dry ingredients, and pumpkin on the wet ingredients and switching to a rubber spatula or wooden spoon, gently fold the ingredients together just until a few streaks of flour remain.
6. Fill jumbo cupcake liners in a jumbo pan 2/3 full of batter. Or use a regular muffin tin.
7. Sprinkle the crumb mixture all over the top of the muffins.
8. Bake for 23-28 minutes and then remove from the oven to cool completely.

9. Sprinkle the tops with powdered sugar and serve.

4. The Softest Pumpkin Rolls

Prep Time: 2hr 5 Minutes

Cook Time: 4hr 15 Minutes

Serving: 32

Ingredients

- 3/4 Cup Sugar
- 1 1/2 Sticks 3/4 Cup Land O'Lakes Unsalted Butter
- 3 Cups Milk Scalded
- 1 Cup Pumpkin Puree
- 1/2 Teaspoon Cinnamon
- 1 Tablespoon Salt
- 4 Eggs
- 1 Tablespoon Yeast Instant, or 2 Tablespoons Regular Yeast. We use instant
- 8-10 Cups Flour
- 1/2 Cup Butter softened, for rolling out rolls.

Instructions

1. Heat a medium sauce pan over medium heat and add the milk.

2. Cook until the edges begin to foam and froth, but do not allow it to boil. There will be a little layer of the milk "skin" on top.

3. Remove from heat and add the sugar, butter, pumpkin, cinnamon and salt.

4. Stir thoroughly and allow to cool to luke warm.

5. Add the yeast, stir and then add the eggs, stirring until they are mixed in.

6. Place the flour in a large bowl.

7. Pour the milk mixture in and stir until the dough has come together, but is still soft. Sometimes we only use like 8 cups of flour and use remaining flour when rolling out the rolls. This is not like a bread dough. It is a slightly sticky dough.

8. Cover the bowl with a towel or saran wrap.

9. Let dough rise for one hour.

10. Push down and divide dough into 2 parts. Heavily flour your work surface using the remaining 1-2 cups of flour and turn the dough out onto the flour. Turn it over so that the flour coats all sides and the dough is no longer sticky.

11. Roll out one portion at a time to 1/2" thick and butter 1/2 of dough with a few pats of butter. Fold the unbuttered dough over the buttered dough and press to seal. Cut into 1" wide strips. Pick up one strip at a time and tie into knots.

12. Or divide into 4 and roll each piece in a circle, butter 2/4 circles and place the unbuttered on top of each one, creating two different buttered, sealed circles. Press down gently and cut into wedges. Starting at the fat end, tightly roll into crescent rolls.

13. Third Option: Cut dough balls, and press each flat. Add a dot of butter and pinch up all of the sides and roll into balls.

14. Place on lightly greased cookie sheet and cover with a towel. Let rise for 1-2 hours more or until doubled in size. Bake at 350 until golden brown, 18-20 min

5. Candied Pecan Bacon Brussels Sprouts

Prep Time: 10 Minutes

Cook Time: 30 Minutes

Serving: 4

Ingredients

- 2 cups Brussel Sprouts ends trimmed off and sliced in half
- 1 tablespoon Johnny's Garlic Spread or other garlic seasoning
- Olive Oil
- 1 tablespoon Butter unsalted
- 1 Cup Candied Pecans
- 3 slices Bacon cooked and chopped
- 1/3-1/2 cup Craisins
- candied pecans
- 3 cups Fisher Nuts pecans
- Fisher Nuts pecans
- 1 Egg White
- 2 teaspoons Water
- 1/2 cup White Sugar

- 1/2 cup Brown Sugar
- 1 tablespoon Cinnamon
- 1 pinch Nutmeg
- 1 pinch Salt

Instructions

For the candied nuts:

1. Preheat the oven to 300 degrees and line a cookie sheet with parchment paper.
2. In a small bowl, whisk together the egg white and water until foamy. Stir into the pecans in a large bowl.
3. Stir in the sugars and seasoning and spread out over the cookie sheet.
4. Bake for 25-27 minutes then allow to cool on the counter all day.
5. For the brussel sprouts
6. Heat a saute pan over medium heat with a drizzle of olive oil and butter.
7. Add the brussel sprouts and stir to coat in the oil mixture.
8. Allow to cook for 5-10 minutes or until tender and golden on the cut side.

9. Add the garlic seasoning (not garlic salt) and cook for an additional minute.

10. Remove to a dish and toss with craisins, bacon and chopped candied pecans.

11. Serve immediately.

6. Sweet Potato Souffle

Prep Time: 1hr 10 Minutes

Cook Time: 1hr 40 Minutes

Serving: 10

Ingredients

- 3 sweet potatoes medium
- 1 egg large
- 1/4 cup butter melted
- pinch salt
- 1/4 cup white sugar
- 1/3 cup brown sugar
- 1/2 teaspoon cinnamon
- 1/2 teaspoon vanilla
- 2 tablespoons milk any milk will do, or heavy cream
- Brown Sugar Pecans
- 1/2 Cup pecans chopped
- 1 Tablespoon Butter
- 1/2 Teaspoon cinnamon
- 1-2 Tablespoons brown sugar
- Topping

- 1/4 cup butter cold and cut in cubes
- 1/2 cup flour
- 1/2 cup brown sugar
- 1/2 teaspoon cinnamon
- 1/2 cup panko bread crumbs

Instructions

1. Preheat the oven to 400 degrees.
2. Place a piece of tin foil on the oven rack.
3. Pierce the sweet potatoes with a fork and bake for 45-60 minutes or until tender.
4. Carefully peel the potatoes and turn the oven down to 350 degrees.
5. Place the sweet potatoes in a large bowl and smash them until smooth.
6. Add the egg, butter, cinnamon, salt, sugars, vanilla and milk.
7. Using a handheld or standing mixer, beat everything together until smooth.
8. Pour the mixture into an 8×9″ baking dish and bake for 30 minutes.
9. Remove from the oven and top with the crumb topping, and bake for an additional 20 minutes.

10. Allow to cool for 5 minutes and serve.

11. Brown Sugar Pecans

12. In a skillet over medium heat, add the pecans and toast evenly for about a minute, tossing often.

13. Add the butter and as it's almost melted, stir in the cinnamon and brown sugar. As soon as things are coated, pour out onto a piece of parchment paper to cool.

14. TOPPING

15. In a medium sized bowl, add the cold butter, flour, sugar and cinnamon.

16. Using a pastry cutter or fork, cut into the mixture until the butter is well incorporated.

17. I like to use my hands at the end.

18. Stir in the panko and pecans and set aside until you're ready to top the casserole.

7. Sausage Stuffing

Prep Time: 20 Minutes

Cook Time: 30 Minutes

Serving: 10

Ingredients

- 12 Cups Country Bread 1 loaf
- 1 Pound Pork Sausage Sage
- 1/3 Cup Butter
- 1 1/2 Cups Red Onion Finely Chopped
- 2 Stalks Celery Chopped
- 5 Cloves Garlic Large, minced
- 1/2 Cup Flat leafed parsley Chopped
- 1 Tablespoon Fresh Sage Chopped
- 1 Tablespoon Fresh Rosemary Chopped
- 2 teaspoons Fresh Thyme Stripped from the stems
- 3/4 teaspoon Sea Salt or more to taste
- 1/2 teaspoon Black Pepper freshly ground
- 1/4 Cup White Cooking Wine (by the vinegar)
- 2 1/4 Cups Chicken Stock low sodium
- 1 Cup Dried Cranberries (optional)

Instructions

1. Preheat the oven to 400°

2. Slice the bread into pieces about 1 inch wide. Place the bread pieces in a single layer on a sheet pan and bake for 5 minutes, or until dried and toasted. Transfer to a very large bowl.

3. Reduce the oven to 350.

4. Meanwhile, in a large saute pan, Cook the sausages over medium heat for about 10 minutes, until browned and cooked through, breaking up the sausage with a fork while cooking. Add to the bread.

5. In the same pan, without draining any grease out, melt the butter and add the onions, celery, garlic, parsley, sage, rosemary or thyme, salt and pepper. Saute over medium heat for 10 minutes, until the vegetables are softened. Add the cooking wine (if using, or sub broth) and allow the to reduce down to half (about 4 minutes).

6. Add the stock and cranberries, stirring well, and pour into the bread. Mix really well with a wooden spoon until all the liquid has been absorbed.

7. Pour the bread stuffing into a 9x12-inch baking dish. Bake for 30 minutes, until browned on top and hot in the middle. Serve warm.

8. The Best Mashed Potatoes

Prep Time: 10Minutes

Cook Time: 35Minutes

Serving: 4

Ingredients

- 2 pounds Russet Potatoes about 6-7 potatoes
- 8 tablespoons Butter melted, plus 2 more for the top
- 1 cup Heavy Cream *half and half or whole milk may be used
- 1 1/2 teaspoons Salt or to taste
- Black pepper to taste

Instructions

1. Place unpeeled potatoes in a large pot (5 Qt+) and cover potatoes with cold water. Never start with hot water or the potatoes will overcook on the outside and be undercooked in the middle.

2. Bring to a boil and cook until easily pierced with a knife, about 20-25 min depending on the size of your potatoes.

3. Drain potatoes well and set aside.

4. Peel the potatoes by sliding the skins off.

5. In a potato ricer, or mesh bowl, push the potatoes through. In the strainer we use a well curved wooden spoon to push them through.

6. Meanwhile, melt the butter in the microwave and warm the cream in a separate bowl. Do NOT mix together.

7. Stir the butter into the potatoes.

8. Add the cream and salt and pepper and stir again until smooth.

9. Serve with additional butter on top!

9. The Most Amazing Apple Pecan Smoked Turkey Breast

Prep Time: 24hrs 5 Minutes

Cook Time: 12hrs 5 Minutes

Serving: 6

Ingredients

For the Smoker:

- Pecan Pellets or chips
- Tin Pan

For the Brine:

- 1/2 Cup Maple Syrup
- 1/4 Cup Brown Sugar
- 1 Cup Kosher Salt
- 4 Cups Apple Juice
- 1 Cup Orange Juice
- 32 ounces Chicken Broth
- 1 Teaspoon Smoked Paprika
- 6.5 lb Turkey Breast bone in
- For the Turkey Rub

- 3 Tablespoons Brown Sugar
- 1 1/2 Tablespoons Smoked Paprika
- 2 Teaspoons Ground Mustard
- 1 Tablespoon Kosher
- 1 Teaspoon Onion Powder
- 1 1/2 Teaspoons Garlic Powder
- 1 Teaspoon Chipotle Chili Pepper Seasoning
- 1 Teaspoon Pepper
- 1 1/2 Teaspoon Cumin
- 6 Tablespoons Butter softened
- 3/4 Cup Pineapple Juice
- 3/4 Cup Water
- For the Gravy
- 1-2 Tablespoon Cornstarch
- 1-2 Tablespoon Water

Instructions

For the Brine:

1. In a large pot, add the brine ingredients. Stir to combine.
2. Rinse the turkey breast thoroughly.

3. Place the turkey in the brine and put the lid on the pot. Refrigerate 10-12 hours or overnight.

4. For the Smoker

5. Remove the turkey from the brine, discarding all liquid and pat the turkey completely dry.

6. In a bowl, combine the spice ingredients and stir to mix.

7. Add the butter and stir again.

8. Rub the mixture all over under and over the skin of the turkey.

9. Heat a Traeger Smoker to 300 degrees with pecan pellets or chips.

10. Place the pineapple juice and water in a tin pan under the rack in the smoker.

11. Put the turkey, breast side down, on the smoker rack and close the lid.

12. Smoke for 3 to 3 1/2 hours depending on your smoker.

13. Remove the turkey to rest for 20 minutes under tented foil, reserving the drippings in the tin pan.

14. Slice the turkey and serve with gravy.

10. The best Potato Rolls

Prep Time: 2hrs 5 Minutes

Cook Time: 15 Minutes

Serving: 32

Ingredients

- 3/4 Cup Sugar
- 1 1/2 Sticks Land O'Lakes Unsalted Butter 3/4 Cup
- 3 Cups Scalded Milk
- 1 Cup Potato Flakes
- 1 Tablespoon Salt
- 4 Eggs
- 1 Tablespoon Instant Yeast or 2 Tablespoons Regular Yeast. We use instant.
- 7 Cups Flour
- 1/3 cup additional butter softened

Instructions

1. Heat a medium sauce pan over medium heat and add the milk.

2. Cook until the edges begin to foam and froth, but do not allow it to boil. There will be a little layer of the milk "skin" on top.

3. Remove from heat and add the sugar, butter, potato flakes and salt.

4. Stir thoroughly and allow to cool to luke warm.

5. Add the yeast, stir and then add the eggs, stirring until they are mixed in.

6. Place the flour in a large bowl.

7. Pour the milk mixture in and stir until the dough has come together, but is still soft. Sometimes we only use like 6- 6 1/2 cups of flour. This is not like a bread dough. It is a slightly sticky dough.

8. Cover the bowl with a towel or saran wrap.

9. Let dough rise for one hour.

10. Push down and divide dough into 2 parts. Roll out one portion at a time to 1/2" thick and butter 1/2 of dough with a few pats of butter. Fold the unbuttered dough over the buttered dough and press to seal. Cut into 1" wide strips. Pick up one strip at a time and tie into knots. Or divide into 4 and roll each piece in a circle, butter 2/4 circles and place the unbuttered on top of each one, creating two different buttered, sealed circles. Press down gently and cut into wedges. Starting

at the fat end, tightly roll into crescent rolls. Place on lightly greased cookie sheet and cover with a towel. Let rise for 1-2 hours more or until doubled in size. Bake at 350 until golden brown, (14-20 min)

11. Instant Pot green Beans and Potatoes

Prep Time: 10 Minutes

Cook Time: 15 Minutes

Serving: 6

Ingredients

- 8 Slices Bacon, chopped
- 1/2 Red Onion, chopped
- 1 Clove Garlic, minced
- 6-8 Potatoes Small Yukon Gold, halved
- 1 Tablespoon Butter
- 2 Pounds Haricot Verts Fresh, trimmed (or Green Beans)
- 3/4 Cup Chicken Broth

Olive Oil

- Salt and Pepper, to taste
- Fresh Parsley, chopped

Instructions

1. Press Saute and 20 minutes on your Instant Pot. Once hot, add the bacon and cook until crisp, stirring occasionally as needed. Remove the bacon to a paper towel lined plate, leaving the grease.
2. Place the onions and garlic in and sauté until tender.
3. Add the potatoes, cut side down and cook until golden, adding a drizzle of olive oil if needed.
4. Add the butter.
5. Throw in the green beans and stir to combine.
6. Add the chicken broth and set it to manual, high pressure for 6 minutes.
7. Allow a natural release and then open the lid, season with salt and pepper to taste and stir in the bacon.
8. Sprinkle the chopped parsley all over the top right before serving.

12. Sweet and Salty Chocolate Caramel Banana Trail Mix

Prep Time: 5 Minutes

Cook Time: 5 Minutes

Serving: 16

Ingredients

- 1 Bag Extra Dark Chocolate Chips
- 1 Bag Snyders Pretzel Rounds
- 1 Bag Kraft Caramel Bits
- 12 ounces Salted Almonds or more to taste
- 2-3 Cups Sweetened Banana Chips broken

Instructions

1. Add all ingredients to a large bowl and toss well. Store in an airtight container for up to 3 weeks.

13. Bakery Style Coffee Cake Muffins

Prep Time: 15 Minutes

Cook Time: 50 Minutes

Serving: 24

Ingredients

For the Streusel:

- 3 Cups Flour
- 1 Cup Brown Sugar
- 1/2 Cup White Sugar
- 1 Teaspoon Kosher Salt
- 2 Tablespoons Cinnamon
- 1 Cup Unsalted Butter (2 sticks= 1 cup)

For the Cake:

- 1/2 Cup Unsalted Butter
- 2 Cups Sugar minus 2 tablespoons
- 1/2 Cup Vegetable Oil
- 2 Eggs large, whisked
- 1 1/2 teaspoons Vanilla Extract
- 4 Cups Flour

- 4 teaspoons Baking Powder

- 1 teaspoon Salt

- 1 Cup Buttermilk

- For the Icing:

- 1 Cup Powdered Sugar

- 1 Teaspoon Vanilla

- 3-4 Tablespoons Heavy Cream (milk is ok)

Instructions

For the Streusel:

2. In a large bowl, stir together the flour, sugars, salt and cinnamon.

3. Melt the butter and allow to cool just slightly so it's still melted but not hot.

4. Stir the butter into the dry ingredients and do not break up clumps unless they are huge. Set aside.

For the Cake:

1. Heat the oven to 350 degrees and line 3 muffin tins with paper liners. These work best when muffins are

involved, see post. See note on muffin tips for the best rise.

2. In a standing mixer, beat the butter and sugar until fluffy, about 1-2 minutes. Add the oil and mix again.

3. Crack in your eggs and add the vanilla and then give the mixer a final turn before dumping in all dry ingredients. Mix until almost incorporated and then add in the buttermilk and stir until barely combined.

4. Make a well in the center of the batter, add about 1 cup of the streusel and cover the streusel with batter.

5. Sprinkle about 1 1/2 cups more streusel on top, and using a rubber spatula, gently fold the clumps of streusel in.

6. Using a cookie scoop, add the batter evenly into each tulip liner and sprinkle generously with streusel.

7. Bake 15-20 minutes, or until a toothpick in the center comes out clean.

8. Allow to cool slightly then drizzle with the icing and serve warm.

14. Pressed Italian Sandwiches

Prep Time: 15Minutes

Cook Time: 6hrs 2Minutes

Serving: 6

Ingredients

- 1 Loaf Italian Bread 12oz, ciabatta or garlic
- 3 oz Prosciutto
- 6 oz Italian Meats Mix (genoa salami, varzi, calabrese)
- 4-6 Slices Tomato
- 2 Red Bell Peppers roasted and seeded, sliced open
- Balsamic Glaze
- Fresh Mozzarella
- 1 Cup Baby Spinach or basil
- 1/4 Cup Pesto

Instructions

1. Slice open the bread and spread one side liberally with pesto. On the other half drizzle a very small amount of olive oil.

2. Lay the tomatoes or roasted red pepper flat. Drizzle with a little balsamic glaze.

3. Layer the meats, cheese and spinach (basil if desired).

4. Close the sandwich and wrap in plastic wrap. Place in the fridge with a heavy skillet or anything very heavy on top for 6 hours or up to overnight.

5. Serve with chips and salad!

15. Buttermilk Biscuits

Prep Time: 10Minutes

Cook Time: 10Minutes

Serving: 12

Ingredients

- 4 Cups All-Purpose Flour Unbleached
- 2 Tablespoons Baking Powder
- 1/2 Teaspoon Baking Soda
- 1 Teaspoon Sugar
- 1 1/2 Teaspoons Salt
- 1 Cup Butter Cold Unsalted, cut into 1/4 inch cubes
- 1 1/2 Cups Buttermilk
- 2 Tablespoons Buttermilk
- 1/4 Cup Melted Butter

Instructions

1. Adjust oven rack to middle and heat to 425.

2. Place the flour, baking powder, baking soda, sugar, and salt in a large bowl or food processor fitted with a metal blade to combine, or whisk in a large bowl.

3. Cut in the butter until it resembles coarse meal with a few slightly larger bumps. Make a well in the center of the flour mixture.

4. Stir in 1 1/2 cups buttermilk with a rubber spatula or fork until just starts to come together then turn out onto a counter top. Knead 3-4 times, but it should still look lumpy.

5. Roll out about 1" thick. Place a 3 1/2" cutter in flour then cut straight up and down through the dough.

6. Arrange with sides of the biscuits touching on a parchment lined baking sheet and brush with the remaining 2 tablespoons buttermilk, bake 8-10 minutes.

7. Remove from the oven and brush with melted butter.

16. Garlic Bread Chicken Parmesan Sandwiches

Prep Time: 10Minutes

Cook Time: 30Minutes

Serving: 4

Ingredients

For the Chicken:

- 2 Tablespoons Olive Oil
- 2 Tablespoons Unsalted Butter
- 2 Chicken Breasts , butterflied
- Seasoned Croutons , crushed
- Jarred Marinara of Choice
- 8 Ounces Mozzarella Sliced
- Parmesan
- Pesto

For the Sandwich:

- 4 Hoagie rolls or French Baguettes
- 1 Stick Unsalted Butter softened

- Garlic Salt with Herbs we prefer Johnny's Garlic Spread from Costco

Instructions

1. Drizzle 2 tablespoons olive oil and place 2 tablespoons of the butter in a large pan and heat to medium high heat.
2. Meanwhile, dredge the chicken in the finely crushed croutons on both sides.
3. Place 2 breasts at a time in the pan and after a minute turn down to medium low. Cook for 5 minutes (consult how to cook chicken in a pan) and flip, cooking another 5-7 minutes or until cooked through to 160 degrees. Remove to a plate, add more butter and oil and repeat with remaining chicken. Set aside.
4. Meanwhile, prepare the pesto.
5. Butter the insides of the bread and sprinkle with garlic salt. Heat the oven to broil and cook open faced until golden. Remove to set aside.
6. Add a spoonful or two of sauce to the bottom bread and place the chicken on top.
7. Cover the chicken in the sauce and add mozzarella.

8. Place under the broiler until the cheese is bubbly, then top with a sprinkle of parmesan cheese and add a smear of pesto to brighten the meal. Top with the other bread and dig in!

17. Tomato Cucumber Salad

Prep Time: 20Minutes

Cook Time: 1hrs 5Minutes

Serving: 6

Ingredients

Salad:

- 8 Small Vine Cocktail Tomatoes (not grape or cherry, but actual vine tomatoes)
- 1 English Cucumber
- 1 Pinch Brown Sugar
- 1/4 Red Onion thinly sliced
- 2 Tablespoons Parsley fresh, chopped
- 2 Tablespoons Cilantro fresh, chopped
- 2 Pinches Salt
- 2 Pinches Pepper

Dressing:

- 1/2 Cup Olive Oil
- 1/4 Cup Red Wine Vinegar
- 1 Squeeze Lemon Juice

- 1 Pinch Pepper
- 1 teaspoon Kosher Salt
- 3 Cloves Garlic minced
- 1 teaspoon Brown Sugar
- 1 teaspoon Dried Basil (or 2 teaspoons fresh, chopped)

Instructions

1. Cut each tomato in 6-8 wedges and then halve them.
2. Trim the ends off of the cucumber and then slice in half lengthwise, creating two pieces. Slice in 1/4" pieces.
3. Toss tomatoes with the brown sugar, onion, and herbs with salt and pepper.
4. In a glass measuring cup, whisk together the dressing ingredients and pour over the tomato salad.
5. Cover in plastic for 1-6 hours on the counter or refrigerate if longer. This is best served the day of and is delicious served with grilled or toasted crostini bread!

18. Glazed lemon snack cake

Prep Time: 10 Minutes

Cook Time: 1hrs 5 Minutes

Serving: 9

Ingredients

Cake:

- 1 1/2 Cups Flour
- 1 Tablespoon Baking Powder
- 1/4 teaspoon Salt
- 3 Lemons zested, reserve lemons for juice
- 3/4 Cup Butter 1 1/2 sticks, softened
- 1/4 Cup Vegetable Oil
- 1 Cup Sugar
- 4 Eggs large, room temperature
- 1/2 Cup Milk
- 2 teaspoons Vanilla
- 1/4 teaspoon Almond Extract
- 2 Tablespoons Lemon Extract
- 2 Tablespoons Lemon Juice
- Lemon Syrup

- 3 Tablespoons Butter
- 3 Tablespoons Sugar
- 4 Tablespoons Lemon Juice
- 1/2 Teaspoon Vanilla

Lemon Icing:

- 1 Cup Powdered Sugar
- 1 1/2 Tablespoons Lemon juice or milk for a very thick and white icing

Instructions

For the Cake:

1. Preheat oven to 350 degrees and line a square 8x8" pan with parchment paper. I like to spray non stick spray on the pan, press in the paper and then spray again.
2. In a large bowl, add the flour, baking powder, salt and lemon zest and whisk to combine.
3. In another large bowl, mix together the butter, oil, sugar, eggs, milk, vanilla, lemon extract, almond extract and lemon juice. Add to the dry ingredients and mix together until no clumps remain.
4. Spread the batter into the lined pan and bake for 45-55 minutes, or until a toothpick comes out clean. While the cake is baking, prepare the lemon syrup.

For the Lemon Syrup:

1. While the cake is baking, add the butter, sugar, lemon juice and vanilla in a small saucepan over medium heat, and stir until melted.
2. Once the cake it done, remove from the oven and prick everywhere with a toothpick. Pour the simple syrup over the top and allow to cool completely (at least 1 hour) before adding the glaze.

For the Lemon Icing:

1. Whisk together powdered sugar and lemon juice. Pour over the cooled cake. Let the cake sit for another hour for the glaze to set up.

19. Garlic Butter Chicken

Prep Time: 2 Minutes

Cook Time: 8 Minutes

Serving: 4

Ingredients

- 6 Chicken Tenders
- 1 1/4 teaspoons Smoked Paprika
- 1/2 teaspoon Poultry Seasoning Montreal chicken works well
- 4 Tablespoons Butter
- 6 Cloves Garlic minced
- 1 teaspoon Italian Seasoning Blend
- 1/2 Cup Cooking White Wine chicken broth or actual white wine
- Salt and Pepper
- 1 1/2 teaspoons Lemon Juice
- Parsley fresh, chopped to garnish

Instructions

2. Season the chicken tenders with smoked paprika, poultry seasoning, salt and pepper. Set aside.

3. Heat a cast-iron skillet on medium high heat and add a good drizzle of olive oil. Add the chicken tenders. Cook for 1-2 minutes or until browning, then turn over and start cooking the other side, about another 2 minutes. Push the chicken tenders to the side of the skillet, away from the high heat.

4. Add the cooking white wine and using a wooden spoon to scrape up any bits and deglaze the pan.

5. Add the butter followed by the garlic and Italian seasoning on top of the chicken tenders and stir to combine well.

6. Add salt if needed and lemon juice and continue to cook the chicken tenders until they are slightly charred on the both sides and cooked through.

7. Add the chopped parsley, stir to combine well. Turn off the heat and serve with an additional squeeze of lemon.

20. Funeral Potatoes

Prep Time: 20 Minutes

Cook Time: 1hrs 5 Minutes

Serving: 8

Ingredients

- 1 can cream of chicken soup
- 2 cups sour cream light
- 1/2 cup butter melted
- 1 teaspoon salt
- 1 teaspoon onion powder
- 1/2 teaspoon garlic powder
- 1/2 Teaspoon pepper
- 24 ounces hash browns frozen squares or shredded
- 2 cups cheddar cheese

Topping:

- 1/2 cup butter unsalted, melted
- 2 1/2 cups Corn Flakes slightly crushed

Instructions

1. Place the potatoes in a colander while you prepare the sauce to defrost them
2. Combine the sour cream, soup and butter in a bowl until smooth. Add in the seasonings and cheese
3. Mix in the frozen hash browns, lifting and folding the mixture until well combined.
4. In a medium bowl, toss the lightly crushed cornflakes with the butter until evenly combined.
5. Scoop out the potato mixture into a 9x13-inch baking dish and top with the buttered cornflakes.
6. Bake at 350 degrees for 45 minutes, until hot and bubbly around the edges.
7. Remove from the oven and let sit for about 10 min and then serve!

21. Savory Beef Pot Pie

Prep Time: 20 Minutes

Cook Time: 2hrs 25 Minutes

Serving: 6

Ingredients

- 1 Puff Pastry 1 full sheet
- 2- 2 1/2 Pounds Beef Roast chopped in 1" pieces

Salt and Pepper:

- 1 Yellow Onion sliced in half horizontally then sliced again so the onion strands are not too long
- 2 Cloves Garlic minced
- 2 Large Carrots peeled and chopped
- 2 Stalks Celery minced
- 1 1/4 Cup Peas frozen
- 1/3 Cup Flour
- 3/4 teaspoon Salt
- 1/4 teaspoon Pepper
- 1 Sprig Rosemary fresh

- 1 teaspoon Thyme Leaves fresh
- 1 3/4 Cups Beef Broth
- 1 Bay Leaf
- 2 Tablespoons Balsamic Vinegar
- 1 Tablespoon Worcestershire Sauce
- 1 teaspoon Dijon Mustard
- 1/3 Cup Whole Milk
- 1 Egg
- 1 Tablespoon Milk

Instructions

1. Heat a large pot or Dutch oven over high heat and add a few tablespoons of olive oil.
2. Dry the meat with paper towels thoroughly then sprinkle generously with salt and pepper. Add the meat to the pot in batches, cooking to brown on each side. Remove to a plate and continue until all meat is browned.
3. Once the meat has been removed, add the onion, celery and carrots. Cook for 5-7 minutes until they begin to soften. Add the garlic, salt and pepper, thyme and rosemary and cook until fragrant, about 1-2 minutes.

4. Stir the flour into the vegetables and cook for 30 seconds then add the meat back into the pot and stir to combine.

5. Gently pour in the beef stock, balsamic, worcestershire sauce, mustard and milk. Stir everything together and bring to a boil. Add the bay leaf. Allow to cook until slightly thickened, about 3-5 minutes.

6. Reduce the heat to low, add the lid and allow to simmer for 90 minutes or until the beef is tender and almost done.

7. Remove the lid and allow to simmer for another 30 minutes until the beef is very tender and the sauce has reduced and thickened slightly.

8. Add the peas and stir them into the meat mixture.

9. Preheat the oven to 425 degrees. Spray a 9x13" casserole dish with nonstick spray and pour in the meat mixture.

10. Unfold the sheet of puff pastry and make a few slits as vents in the top of the pie. Place the puff pastry on top of the filling. Whisk the egg wash of egg and milk together and brush gently over the puff pastry.

11. Bake at 425 degrees for 30 minutes and enjoy!

22. Creamy Sausage and Peppers over Mashed Potatoes

Prep Time: 5 Minutes

Cook Time: 25 Minutes

Serving: 4

Ingredients

- 1 pound Italian sausage links 1 package
- 1 small green pepper sliced
- 1 small red pepper sliced
- 1 small yellow onion sliced thin
- 2 Tablespoons cooking white wine
- 1 can fire roasted diced tomatoes
- 6 ounces tomato paste
- 8 ounces tomato sauce
- 12 ounces water
- ½ teaspoon Italian seasoning
- 1 teaspoon sugar
- ½ teaspoon salt
- 1/3 cup heavy cream
- Parmesan Cheese for finishing

- mashed potatoes

Instructions

1. Get the potatoes boiling before you get started on the sausage and peppers so that they are ready to mash as the sausage and peppers simmer.
2. Heat a tablespoon of olive oil in a large skillet over medium-high heat.
3. Brown sausages on all sides, until almost cooked through, remove and cut into ¼ inch slices. You don't have to worry about cooking them all the way through as they will finish cooking while the sauce simmers.
4. In the same pan drizzle another teaspoon or so of olive oil and sauté the peppers and onions until slightly softened, about five minutes.
5. Return sausage back to the pan and deglaze with white wine.
6. Add diced tomatoes, tomato paste, tomato sauce, water, Italian seasoning, sugar, salt and heavy cream.
7. Stir to combine.
8. Bring to a boil and then reduce to a simmer.
9. Simmer for ten minutes. As the sauce simmers, drain the potatoes and mash them.

10. Season with salt and pepper and garnish with grated parmesan cheese.
11. Serve over the mashed potatoes.

23. Southern Macaroni and Cheese

Prep Time: 15 Minutes

Cook Time: 30 Minutes

Serving: 6

Ingredients

- 16 Ounces Elbow Macaroni
- 3 1/2 Cups Sharp Cheddar Cheese shredded (reserve 1 cup for topping)
- 1/4 Cup Butter softened
- 1 1/2 Cups Milk whole or 2%
- 3 Eggs beaten
- 1/2 Cup Sour Cream
- 1/2 Teaspoon Salt

Carrian's Extra GOOEY Version:

- 16 Ounces Elbow Macaroni see note
- 2 Cups Heavy Cream
- 1 Cup and Half or whole milk
- 7 Tablespoons Butter melted
- 2 Large Eggs whisked in a bowl

- 3 Tablespoons Sour Cream
- 1 1/4 Teaspoon Season Salt see note
- 1/2 Teaspoon Garlic Powder
- 1/2 Teaspoon Onion Powder
- 1 Teaspoon Salt
- 1/4 Teaspoon Pepper
- 16 Ounces Colby Jack Cheese shredded, Tillamook works best
- 8 Ounces Monterey Jack Cheese shredded
- 8 Ounces Sharp Cheddar Cheese shredded

Instructions

1. Preheat oven to 350 degrees and spray a 9x11" casserole dish.
2. Cook the macaroni per package instructions.
3. Place the pasta in a large bowl and while still hot and add 2 1/2 cups cheese and butter.
4. In a medium bowl, combine the remaining ingredients, whisking to combine, and add to the macaroni mixture.
5. Pour macaroni mixture into a casserole dish, top with remaining 1 cup of cheese and bake for 30 to 45 minutes.
6. Serve immediately.

7. Carrian's Version

8. Heat the oven to 375 degrees

9. Butter a 9x13 (or 8x8 works but it will be piled very high) dish and set aside.

10. Heat a pot of water to boiling and add 2 teaspoons salt and the pasta. Cook until al dente and drain. Meanwhile, melt the butter and set aside.

11. In a large bowl, add the pasta and toss evenly with the butter, mixing thoroughly before moving on.

12. Add the cream, half and half and eggs and mix thoroughly again. Add the seasonings and stir to combine.

13. In a large bowl, toss together the Colby jack and Monterey jack cheese. Sprinkle in 16 ounces and stir together. Add the sharp cheese and gently fold it all together.

14. Spread the mixture into the pan and sprinkle the remaining cheese all over the top. Bake for 35 minutes and then set out to rest for 5 minutes before serving.

24. Sweet Potato Souffle

Prep Time: 1hrs 5 Minutes

Cook Time: 1hrs 50 Minutes

Serving: 10

Ingredients

3 sweet potatoes medium:

- 1 egg large
- 1/4 cup butter melted

pinch salt:

- 1/4 cup white sugar
- 1/3 cup brown sugar
- 1/2 teaspoon cinnamon
- 1/2 teaspoon vanilla
- 2 tablespoons milk any milk will do, or heavy cream
- Brown Sugar Pecans
- 1/2 Cup pecans chopped
- 1 Tablespoon Butter
- 1/2 Teaspoon cinnamon
- 1-2 Tablespoons brown sugar

Topping:

- 1/4 cup butter cold and cut in cubes
- 1/2 cup flour
- 1/2 cup brown sugar
- 1/2 teaspoon cinnamon
- 1/2 cup panko bread crumbs

Instructions

1. Preheat the oven to 400 degrees.
2. Place a piece of tin foil on the oven rack.
3. Pierce the sweet potatoes with a fork and bake for 45-60 minutes or until tender.
4. Carefully peel the potatoes and turn the oven down to 350 degrees.
5. Place the sweet potatoes in a large bowl and smash them until smooth.
6. Add the egg, butter, cinnamon, salt, sugars, vanilla and milk.
7. Using a handheld or standing mixer, beat everything together until smooth.
8. Pour the mixture into an 8×9″ baking dish and bake for 30 minutes.

9. Remove from the oven and top with the crumb topping, and bake for an additional 20 minutes.

10. Allow to cool for 5 minutes and serve.

11. Brown Sugar Pecans

12. In a skillet over medium heat, add the pecans and toast evenly for about a minute, tossing often.

13. Add the butter and as it's almost melted, stir in the cinnamon and brown sugar. As soon as things are coated, pour out onto a piece of parchment paper to cool.

Topping:

1. In a medium sized bowl, add the cold butter, flour, sugar and cinnamon.

2. Using a pastry cutter or fork, cut into the mixture until the butter is well incorporated.

3. I like to use my hands at the end.

4. Stir in the panko and pecans and set aside until you're ready to top the casserole.

25. The best Pork Carnitas

Prep Time: 8hrs 5 Minutes

Cook Time: 12hrs 5 Minutes

Serving: 16

Ingredients

Brine:

- 1 1/2 Cups Orange Juice
- 1/2 Cup Pineapple juice or lemon juice
- 20 cloves garlic
- 2 Cups apple cider Vinegar
- 1/2 Cup Brown Sugar
- 2 teaspoons sea Salt
- 1 Tablespoon Cumin
- 1 Tablespoon Oregano
- 1 Tablespoon Orange Peel dried
- 1 Tablespoon Smoked Paprika
- 1 Tablespoon Chili Powder
- 1/2 cup oil
- Pork Rub
- 3-4 lb Pork Butt or shoulder , bone-in

- 2 Tablespoons Cumin
- 1 Tablespoon Oregano
- 1 1/2 Teaspoons Orange Peel dried
- 2 Teaspoons Garlic Powder
- 1 Teaspoon Ground Coriander

Cooking:

Canola Oil, for final crisping

- 1/2 Cup Orange Juice
- 1/4 Cup Lime Juice
- 1/4 Cup Chicken Broth

Instructions

For the Brine:

1. Combine all brine ingredients in a blender and blend until smooth. Heat the oil in a pan over medium heat. Remove from heat and then add the blender sauce, stirring carefully so it doesn't hop and splatter.
2. Spread over the pork and place a lid on then stick it in the fridge for 8 hours or overnight.

For the Pork:

1. Heat the oven to 225 degrees F.

2. Remove the pork from the brine and pat dry with paper towels, reserving the marinade.
3. Mix the rub together and rub all over the pork.
4. Mix together the liquids from the "cooking section" and pour in the bottom of the roasting pan.
5. Add the pork, then pour the marinade over the top again.
6. Cook for 12-14 hours or until internal temperature reaches 200 degrees F.
7. Remove the meat and let rest for up 2 hours.
8. Shred the meat and place the liquids in a fat separator.
9. Heat some oil in a pan over medium high heat.
10. Add the shredded pork in small amounts and toss as it begins to crisp. Remove to a pan and repeat until all batches are done.
11. Toss with a little of the juices from the fat separator and serve!

26. Skillet Italian Sausage and Peppers with Whole-Wheat Penne

Prep Time: 5 Minutes

Cook Time: 25 Minutes

Serving: 4

Ingredients

- 12 ounces whole-wheat penne pasta
- 1 pound Italian sausage links 1 package
- 1 small green pepper sliced
- 1 small red pepper sliced
- 1 small yellow onion sliced thin
- ½ cup red wine we use cooking red wine
- 6 ounces tomato paste
- 8 ounces tomato sauce
- 12 ounces water
- ½ teaspoon Italian seasoning
- 1 teaspoon sugar
- ½ teaspoon salt
- Parmesan Cheese for finishing

Instructions

1. In a large pot of salted water, cook pasta until al dente.

2. Reserve starchy cooking water.

3. Heat a tablespoon of olive oil in a large skillet over a medium-high heat.

4. Brown sausages on all sides, until almost cooked through, remove and cut into ¼ inch slices. You don't have to worry about cooking them all the way through, they will finish cooking while the sauce simmers.

5. In the same pan drizzle another teaspoon or so of olive oil and sauté the peppers and onions until slightly softened, about five minutes.

6. Return sausage back to the pan and deglaze with red wine.

7. Add tomato paste, tomato sauce, water, Italian seasoning, sugar and salt.

8. Stir to combine.

9. Bring to a boil and then reduce to a simmer.

10. Simmer for ten minutes.

11. Add penne to the skillet, toss with sauce. If needed add starchy pasta water to loosen the sauce up.

12. Season with salt and pepper and garnish with grated parmesan cheese.

27. Instant Pot Award Winning Chili

Prep Time: 10 Minutes

Cook Time: 40 Minutes

Serving: 8

Ingredients

- 1 1/2 Pounds Ground Beef
- 6 Strips of Bacon good quality, chopped
- 1 Can Kidney Beans 15 ounces, drained
- 1 Can Pinto Beans 15 ounces, drained
- 1 Can Black beans 15 ounces, drained
- 1 Can Fire Roasted Diced tomatoes 15 ounces, with juice
- 1 Can Tomato Paste 6 ounce
- 1 Red Onion chopped
- 1 Red Bell Pepper seeded and chopped
- 1 Jalapeño seeded and minced *optional
- 2 Cups Beef Stock
- 1 Tablespoon Dried Oregano
- 2 Teaspoons Ground Cumin
- 2 Teaspoons Kosher Salt

- 1 Teaspoon Ground Black Pepper
- 1 Teaspoon Smoked Paprika
- 2 Tablespoons Chili Powder
- 1 Tablespoon Worcestershire Sauce
- 1 Tablespoon Garlic minced

For Garnish:

- Sour Cream
- Cilantro
- Cheese shredded

Instructions

1. Turn your instant pot to sauté and add the bacon.
2. Cook until crisp, stirring often to cook evenly.
3. Remove the bacon to a paper towel lined plate.
4. Add the onions and peppers and cook until tender.
5. Add the meat and cook until browned.
6. Drain off any excess grease, we just tilt the pot and use a large spoon.
7. Add all of the remaining ingredients and 3/4 of the bacon and stir to combine.
8. Turn the instant pot to chili (if you don't have a "chili" setting, use the "manual" setting) and cook for 18-20

minutes*. Allow pressure to release for 10-15 minutes or quick release with the vent.

9. Serve with limes, sour cream, cheese, and a little bacon!

28. Cheesy Southwestern Chicken Tortilla Soup

Prep Time: 30 Minutes

Cook Time: 30 Minutes

Serving: 6

Ingredients

- 3 Chicken Breasts
- 15 Ounce Tostitos Salsa Con Queso
    - oz Soup cream of potato, (1 standard can)
- 1 Cup Sour Cream
- 1 3/4 Cups Chicken Broth (or 1 14.5 ounce can)
- 2 oz Green Chiles fire roasted diced,
- 2 Cups Frozen Corn
- 1 Packet Taco Seasoning
- 1/4 Cup Chopped Fresh Cilantro, plus more for garnish
- Tostitos Scoops Chips

Instructions

1. Preheat the oven to 350 degrees F.

2. Sprinkle salt and pepper on each side of the chicken and place in a baking dish.

3. Cover with foil and bake for 30 minutes.

4. Remove from the oven, and using two forks, shred the meat and set aside.

5. In a large pot over medium heat, add the salsa con queso, cream of potato soup, sour cream and chicken broth. Whisk to combine.

6. Switch to a wooden spoon and stir in the chills, corn, taco seasoning, cilantro and chicken.

7. Bring to a simmer and serve or keep on low for an hour or two.

8. Serve with Tostitos Scoops chips.

9. Store in a plastic container, sealed in the fridge for up to 1 week. Do not freeze.

29. Chicken Pot Pie

Prep Time: 20 Minutes

Cook Time: 1hrs 50 Minutes

Serving: 8

Ingredients

For the Crust:

- 2 1/2 Cup All-Purpose Flour
- 1 Cup Unsalted Butter very cold, cut into 1/2-inch cubes (2 sticks)
- 1 Teaspoon Salt
- 1 Teaspoon Granulated Sugar
- 8-12 Tablespoon Ice Water

For the filling:

- 1 Rotisserie Chicken , meat removed and cut into cubes, see note
- 1 Cup Carrots , chopped
- 1 Cup Frozen Corn
- 1 Cup Frozen Peas
- 1/3 Cup Unsalted Butter

- 1/2 Yellow Onion , minced

- 1 Stick Celery , sliced

- 2 Cloves Garlic , minced

- 1/3 Cup All-Purpose Flour

- 3/4 Teaspoon Salt

- 1/4 Teaspoon Pepper

- 1 Pinch Nutmeg

- 1 Teaspoon Fresh Thyme

- 1 3/4 Cup Chicken Broth

- 2/3 Cup Whole Milk (or heavy cream for an extra creamy pot pie)

For the Egg Wash:

- 1 Egg

- 1 Teaspoon Water

Instructions

For the Crust:

1. Place the flour, sugar and salt into a bowl and mix well.

2. Add the butter and using a pastry cutter or two forks, mix until the butter is pea sized.

3. Add the water, just a few tablespoons at a time, stirring gently with a fork until the dough is just coming

together but is still crumbly. Test that the dough is ready by squeezing the dough in your hands until it holds.

4. Smash the dough together and separate into two balls.

5. Wrap in plastic wrap and rest in the fridge for 1 hour. Allow to sit out for a few minutes and then roll out dough.

6. Preheat the oven to 425 degrees F.

7. Roll out half of the dough into the pie plate. Set pie plate and remaining dough in plastic wrap in the fridge.

8. For the Filling:

9. Place the carrots, corn and peas in a pan with just enough water to cover them. Heat over medium heat until soft, about 15 minutes. Drain.

10. Stir together the chicken and veggies in a bowl. Set aside.

11. In a large dutch oven or pot, add the butter and once melted add the onions, celery and garlic, cooking until translucent, about 3 minutes.

12. Stir in flour and seasonings, and herbs. Cook, stirring continuously for 30 seconds.

13. Slowly add the broth and milk, stirring frequently until thick. Remove from heat.

14. Stir in the chicken and veggies and pour into a pie dish.

15. Roll the remaining pie crust over the top and pinch the edges shut. Cut slits in the top of the pie.

16. Whisk together the egg and the water and brush it all over the top crust.

17. Bake for 30 minutes at 425 degrees F, or until golden brown.

18. Allow to cool slightly and serve!

30. Flank Steak

Prep Time: 8hrs 10 Minutes

Cook Time: 15 Minutes

Serving: 4

Ingredients

- 2 lbs flank steak
- 1/2 cup soy sauce
- 1/3 cup vegetable oil
- 2 tablespoons dark brown sugar
- 1/4 cup Worcestershire sauce
- 1 teaspoon dijon mustard
- 4 cloves garlic medium, minced
- 2 tablespoons chives minced, fresh
- 1 1/2 teaspoons ground pepper
- 2 teaspoons balsamic vinegar

Instructions

1. Mix all ingredients together in a ziploc or a large dish.

2. Add the flank steak and marinate (covered) in the fridge overnight or at least all day.

3. Heat the gas grill to high heat. Remove the steak from the marinade and lay on the grill for 2 minutes per side. Then turn down to medium and cook another 7-10 minutes, flipping halfway again, or until an internal temperature of 130 for medium rare, or longer for medium etc. Remove and set aside to rest on a cutting board with foil draped over the top.

4. Meanwhile, place 1/2 of the remaining marinade in a sauce pan over medium heat.

5. Bring the marinade to a simmer for 10 minutes, set aside.

6. Slice the steak against the grain and serve with a drizzle of additional sauce if desired